I0415330

H_2O

Workouts®

Basic Moves

Francine Milford, LMT

H2O Workouts®: Basic Moves by Francine Milford, LMT

ISBN: 978-1-105-82210-0

Caution: Please consult your physician or health care provider before beginning this or any other exercise program.

Chapter One
Fitness for the Next Generation

As more people recognize the need to live healthier lives, they have begun to set goals on how they will achieve and maintain a healthy body through proper nutrition and balanced work schedules.

Soon, many people were experiencing injuries from pushing their bodies too long and too far. When people are impatient to see results, they tend to exercise for long hours in a short period of time. Overuse injuries is one of the most common injuries found in the fitness industry, and no one is immune from the dangers of injury.

But one exercise route sets its self apart from the others-water exercise. Water is the best exercise for all body types and fitness levels.

I call the water environment, the Great Equalizer. When I have taught water aerobic classes I would have ladies enter the water on crutches and even one came to class in a wheelchair. Once in the water, you could not tell the ladies apart.

In the water environment, everyone is equal and everyone can receive a workout that is right for them and their fitness level. In this book I will list exercises in **LEVELS**. If you are a beginner, then please stick to **Level One** exercises. As your body becomes familiar with the moves and becomes stronger, then move on up to **Level Two** and **Level Three**.

Principles of Water

The water environment offers two important natural occurring effects to the water routine: *buoyancy* and *resistance*.

Buoyancy is the property of water that allows you the ability to float and to keep objects afloat; in this case, that object is you. This acts as a cushion and in so doing, it protects you joints from injury, strain and re-injury. Many rehabilitation centers use the water environment in their treatment sessions.

While in the water environment, people can perform exercises they otherwise could not on land. Among these exercises are jumps, leaps, jumping jacks and pivots.

Amazingly enough, the ability of water to be buoyant also allows water to provide resistance to water aerobics. Through changing direction, adding speed, or using longer levers, the water can provide a complete and thorough workout. The water environment can become a natural total body workout. The more you put into your workout, the more you will receive from it. The faster you move, the harder the exercise becomes. Water aerobics provide a safe alternative to the land aerobic class.

Water aerobics is also the perfect environment for those who are overweight or suffer from physical injuries. When you stand in water that is chest deep, you weigh only 10% of your normal body weight.

In water where you cannot touch the bottom of the pool, you will receive a total non impact workout. (Be sure to wear a flotation device if you are planning on doing deep water exercises.)

The water environment is also a great place to practice your golf or tennis swing. Even dancers and weight trainers can use the resistance in the water to build up muscles in a safe way.

Preparing to get Wet

When beginning your water exercise routine, the most important consideration is your swim suit. Find a suit that will cling comfortably to your body and still allow you freedom of movement. Stay away from suits that will quickly fill with water with each jump that you take or that will ride up with each kick. If a suit isn't comfortable you will be fussing more with the suit than you will be concentrating on the exercises.

Tips for a Safe Workout

Do's and Dont's
- Do wear aqua shoes or aqua socks.
- Do keep head in alignment with the spine.
- Do exercise in water that is of correct depth.
- Do breathe slowly and deeply.
- Drink plenty of water before during and after your exercise routine.
- Do work at your own fitness level
- Do consult with your doctor before beginning this exercise program.
- Stop exercising if you feel faint, dizzy, nausea, or shortness of breath.
- Don't smoke or drink alcohol while doing exercises.
- Don't make fast, uncontrolled movements of the head or trunk in any direction.
- Don't use extreme range of motion.
- Don't use quick, jerky movement.
- Don't exercise with food or gum in your mouth.
- If you feel tired-stop

Chapter Two
The Warm-up

As in any exercise program, it is important to prepare the body for the work that you are planning to put it through. We call this preparation, the Warm-Up.

In the Warm-Up you will increase the flow of blood to each and every muscle of the body. In this way, you will greatly reduce the risk of injury.

Warm-up exercises are usually gentle and slow activities that normally last 5 to 15 minutes. During this phase all the muscles and joints should be put through simple movements beginning with small range of motions and then increasing to larger, or full, range of motion.

In a typical land aerobic or workout class, we begin simply with marching in placing. The same holds true for water aerobics. In this chapter we will include several muscle groups that you will need to be sure you warm-up before beginning a water aerobics class. For some, this may be all the exercise that you can do in one day and if so, that is perfectly ckay. What is important is that you move and stretch your body as often as you can throughout the day to keep it limber and lubricated.

Following a 3 to 5 minute warm-up exercise (such as marching in place) you could do some of the following walking exercises for the next 20-45 minutes:

- Walk forward and backwards
- Walk to the right and walk to the left
- Walk sideways to the right and left
- Walk in a big clockwise circle, and then counter clockwise.
- Walk on your toes
- Walk on your heels
- Walk like a crab sideways bouncing from flat feet with knees bent.
- Walk forward and backward while you punch the water.
- Do your favorite Western Two Step.
- Alternate between fast and slow walking.
- Do the Soldier Walk, known on Goose Stepping
- Walk doing knee lifts forward and front leg lift backwards
- Do Pendulum Swings with your legs side to side
- Do the Rocking Horse
- Do Hamstring Curls forward and backwards.
- Do the Waltz, Salsa, Tango, etc.

The Toe and Ankle Warm-up

Some warm-up exercises and stretches can be performed inside, or at poolside.

1. Toe and Ankle

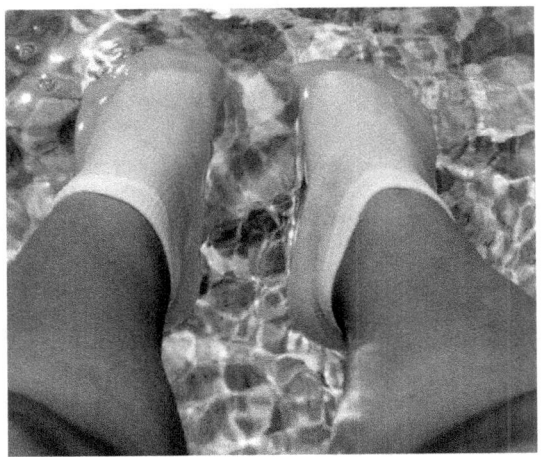

To Do: Slowly point your toes. Hold and release. You will also feel a stretch in the front part of your leg, this is the anterior tibialis. When this muscle is not properly warmed up and stretched, many people suffer from Shin splints. The front of your leg should begin to feel warm. Repeat this stretch for eight repetitions.

2. Toe and Ankle

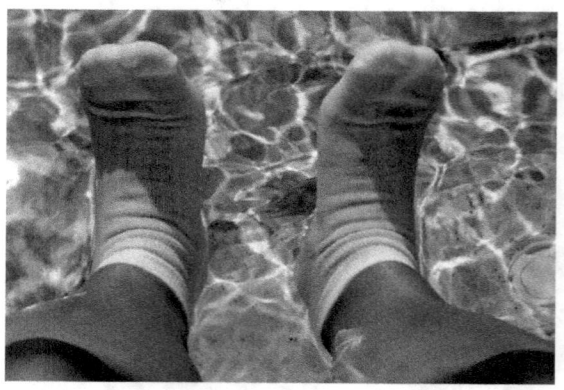

To Do:
Flex your toes by pulling your toes towards you as far as you comfortably can. Hold and release. Feel the stretch from each toe as your attempt to bring each toe towards you and then release it.

Feel the stretch in your Achilles heel and lower calf muscle. Do not strain through this stretch. Do for eight repetitions.

3. Toes and Ankle

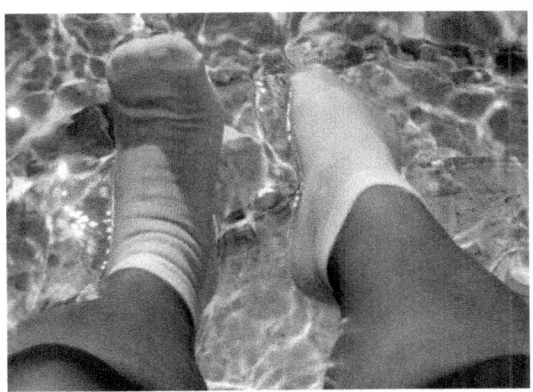

To Do:
Press your right toes away from your body while you bring your left toes toward you body, hold for a few seconds, and then relax the stretch. Now, bring your right towed toward your body and press your left toes away from your body at the same time.

Continue to alternate between your two feet in this way for a total of eight repetitions.

4. Toe and Ankle

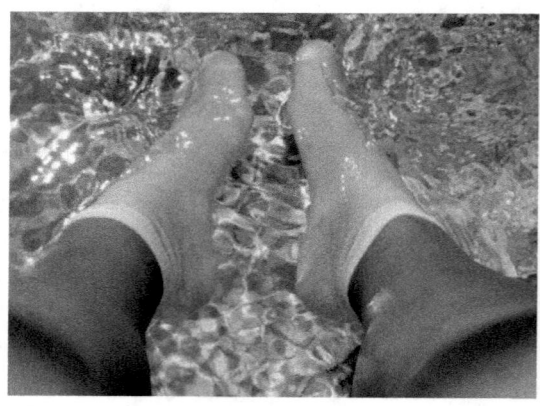

To Do:
In the exercise above you will press the soles of
your feet towards each other, hold for a few
seconds, and then relax the stretch. Perform this
stretch for eight repetitions.

Now, press the soles of your feet away
from each other.
Repeat for a total of eight repetitions.

5. Toe and Ankle
Feet Swinging

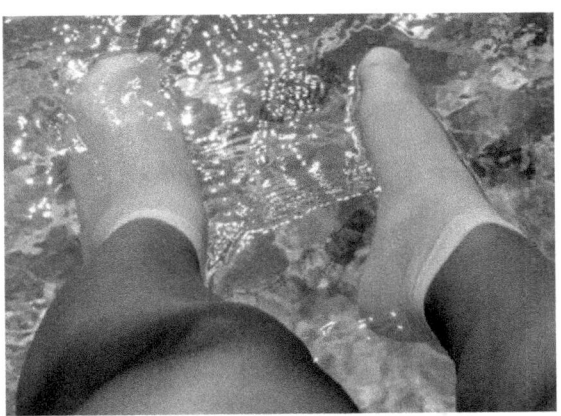

To Do:
In the exercise above you will swing both of your feet to your right and hold for a few seconds. Then swing both of your feet to the left, hold for a few seconds, and then relax.

Perform these feet swinging exercises for eight repetitions. The trick is to swing your feet only-not your legs.

Have fun with the exercise feeling the resistance of the water on your feet. Relax and enjoy.

6. Toes and Ankles
Circles

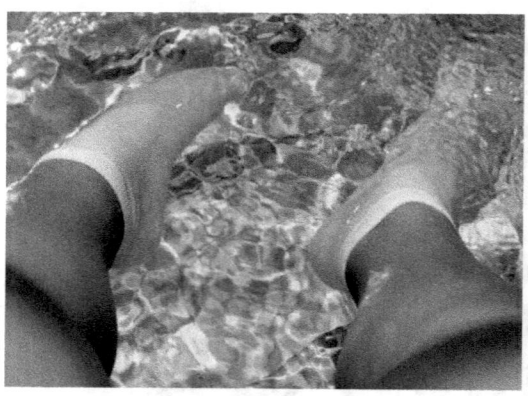

To Do:
Using both feet at the same time, begin to make move your feet in a circle moving clockwise. Begin by making eight small circles and then continue to enlarge each circle until you are making eight of the largest circles you can with you feet.

Now, repeat the same exercise this time creating the smallest circles we can with both feet moving in a counter clockwise movement, enlarging the circles until we are able to make eight of the largest counter clockwise circle we can.

Warm-ups for the Neck

Like the warm-ups for the toes and ankles, warm-ups for the neck can be performed on land before you enter the water environment. Do not push these stretches beyond what your physical capabilities are. Stretches should not be painful. If they are, stop and consult with your health care provider.

Starting Position

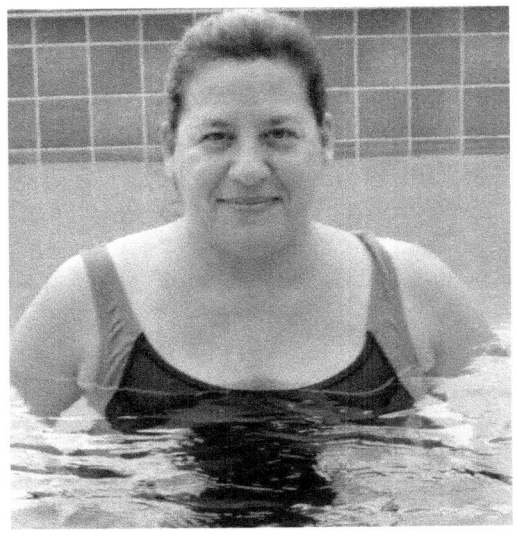

Neck Warm-ups

1-Neck

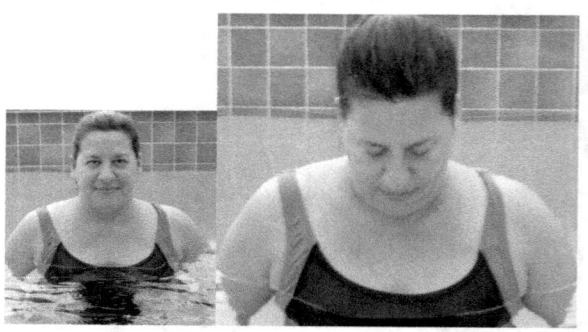

To Do:
Inhale. As you exhale, slowly allow your head to fall forward touching your chin to your chest. Slowly inhale and return your head to the starting position. Repeat for eight repetitions.

2-Neck

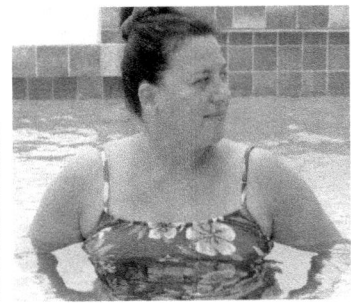

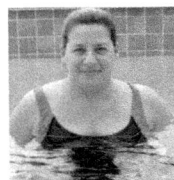

To Do:
Inhale. As you exhale, slowly turn your head to left aligning your chin to over your left shoulder Slowly inhale and as you exhale, begin to return your head to the starting position. Do for eight repetitions and repeat exercise on looking right.

3-Neck

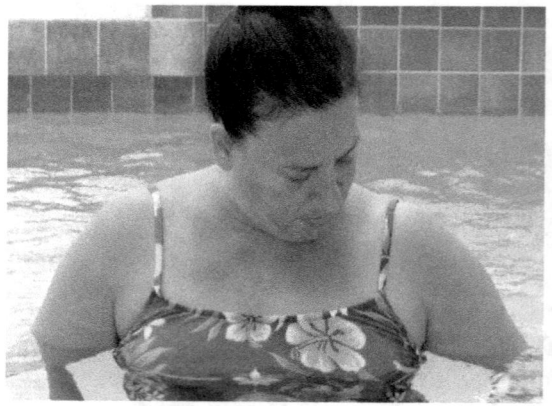

To Do:
Inhale. As you exhale, slowly allow your chin to drop to the left to a point that is located half way between the center of your chest and your left shoulder (note: if you cannot touch your chin to your chest, this is alright, don't force the movement.) Slowly inhale and as you exhale, begin to return your head to the starting position. Repeat eight times. Repeat exercise on the right side.

4-Neck

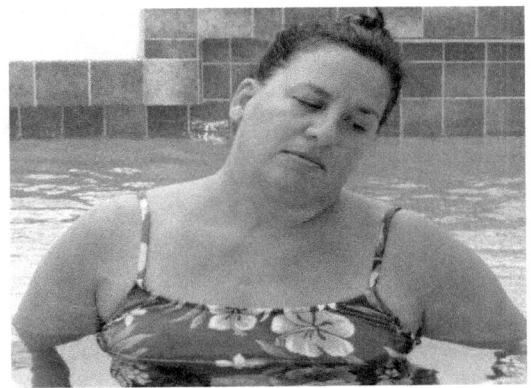

To Do:
Inhale. As you exhale, slowly allow your left ear to drop to your left shoulder (note: if you cannot touch your ear to your shoulder, this is alright, don't force the movement.) Slowly inhale and as you exhale, begin to return your head to the starting position. Repeat eight times before performing this exercise on the other side of your body.

5-Neck
Head Rolls

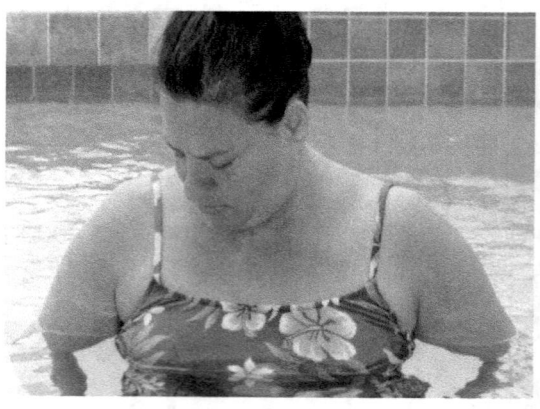

To Do:
Imagine your nose is the hands of a clock. The numbers of the wall clock are right in front of your face.

Inhale and as you slowly exhale moving clockwise in a circle. Repeat for eight repetitions. Repeat the exercise, this time moving counter-clockwise. Repeat for eight repetitions.

Shoulders Warm-ups

1-Shoulders

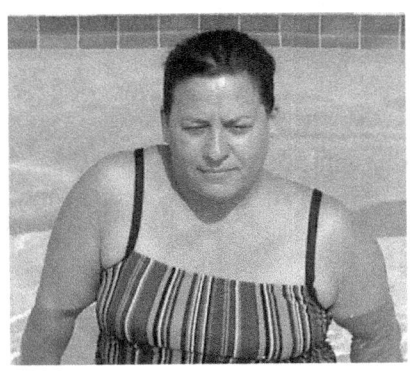

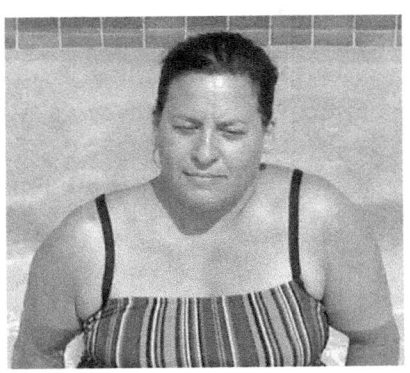

To Do:
Begin by planting both feet flat on the bottom of the pool. Bend your knees slightly and arms down at your sides.

Now, standing perfectly straight, inhale and bring your right shoulder up to your right ear and hold. As you exhale release the shoulder back down to starting position. Remember - do NOT bring your ear down to meet the shoulder. This is very important. Repeat for a total of eight repetitions. Now, inhale and bring your left shoulder up to your left ear and hold. As you exhale, relax and return to the starting position. Repeat for a total of 8 repetitions.

Alternating Shoulders: Inhale and bring your right shoulder up to your right ear and hold. Exhale and relax the shoulder back to the starting position. Inhale and bring your left shoulder up to your left ear and hold. Exhale and relax the shoulder back to the starting position. Repeat for a total of 16 repetitions. Do NOT bring ears to shoulders.

2-Shoulders
Shrugs

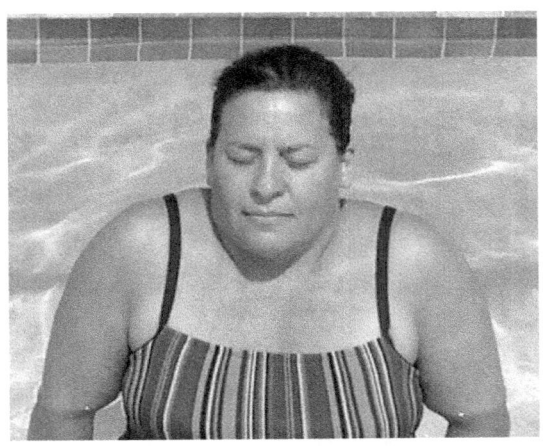

To Do:
Inhale and bring both of your shoulders up to your ears and hold for a few seconds. Exhale and allow both shoulders to relax and return to the starting position. Continue for a total of 16 repetitions.

3-Shoulders
Circles

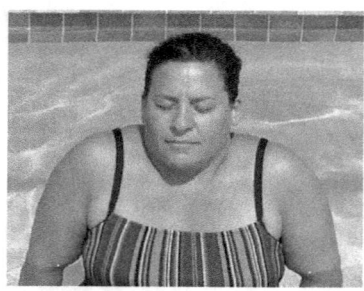

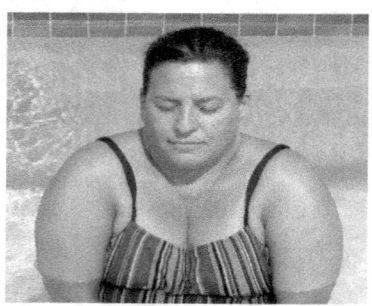

To Do: Inhale and bring both shoulders up to your ears and as you exhale allow the shoulders to push forward, then down, then back behind you forming a circle. Do eight times in one direction, then eight times in the other.

Warm-up for the Wrists

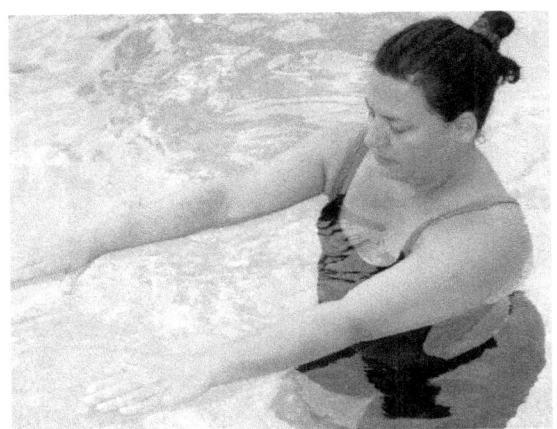

Starting Position

To Do:

Starting Position:
Begin in the starting position. Extend both of your arms straight out in front of your body with fingers pointing away from your body. This is the starting position.

1. Wrists

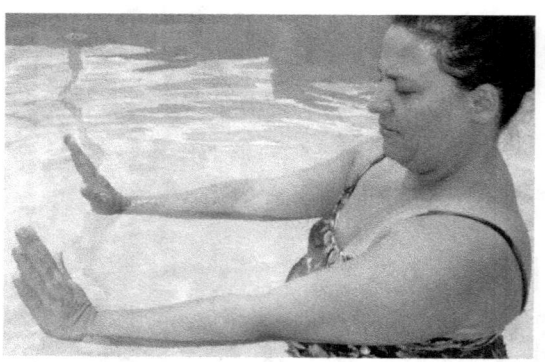

To Do:
Take a nice slow, deep breath and at the same time lift the fingers of both of your hands towards you while keeping the heel of your hand pushing away from your body, hold the stretch for a few seconds. As you slowly exhale, lower your fingers back to the starting position. Repeat for a total of eight repetitions.

2. Wrists

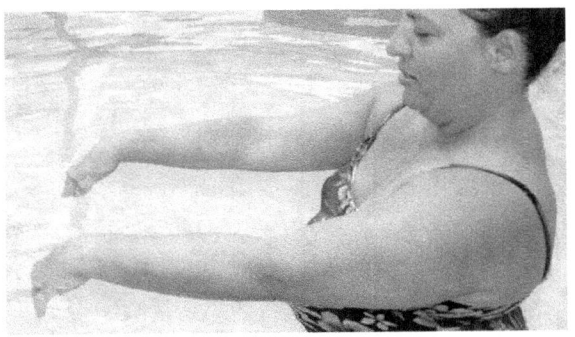

To Do:
Extend both of your arms straight out in front of your body. Do not lock your elbows. If this is uncomfortable, just relax your arms and dc the best that you can.

Inhale and point the fingers of both of your hands down towards the bottom of the pool, while keeping your arms extended away from your body, hold the stretch for a few seconds.

As you slowly exhale, raise your fingers back to the starting position as shown in the picture above, on the left. Repeat for a total of eight repetitions.

3. Wrists

Starting Position

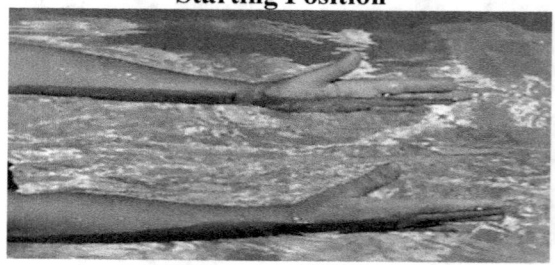

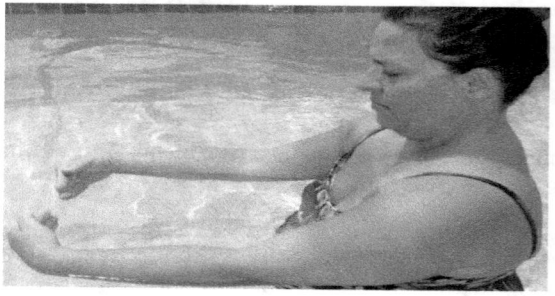

To Do: Extend both of your arms straight out in front of your body. Take a deep breath and point the fingers of both of your hands towards each other. Hold the stretch for a few seconds. Exhale and lower your fingers back to the starting position. Repeat for a total of eight repetitions.

4. Wrists

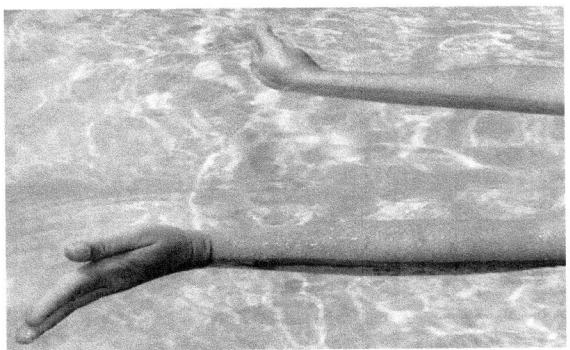

To Do:
Extend both of your arms straight out in front of your body. Take a breath and at the same time, point the fingers of both of your hands away from each other while keeping your arms extended straight in front of your body, hold the stretch for a few seconds. As you slowly exhale, return your fingers back to the starting position. Repeat for a total of eight repetitions.

5. Wrists
Circles

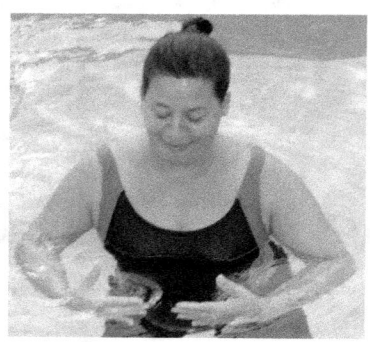

To Do:
Extend both of your arms straight out in front of your body. Begin with your fingers facing each other as shown in the picture above. Make outward circles with your wrists. (The right hand will be making clockwise circles and the left hand will be making counter clockwise circles at the same time.) Do for eight repetitions. Reverse the direction. Do for eight repetitions. You should feel nice warmth in your wrists with this exercise. Great after a day of typing or craft work.

6. Wrist and Forearm

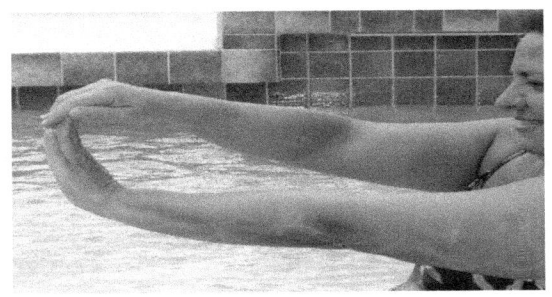

To Do:
Extend your left arm straight out from the front of your body with your fingers pointed upward.

Extend your right arm straight out from the front of your body on top of your left arm and gently grab on to the fingers of your left hand.

Now, take a nice slow deep breath in. As you exhale, gently apply pressure to the fingers of the left hand pressing them toward the front of your body; hold the stretch for a few seconds, then release.

Repeat the exercise for a total of eight repetitions. Do not over stretch.

7. Wrist and Forearm

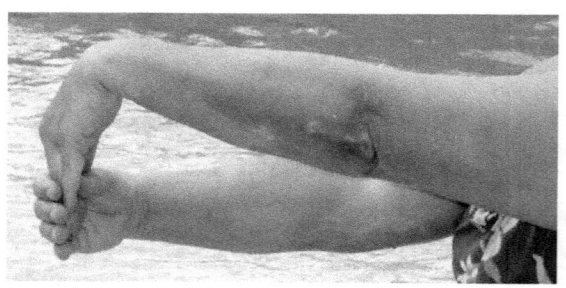

To Do:
Extend your left arm straight out from the front of your body with your fingers pointed down towards the bottom of the pool.

Extend your right arm straight out from the front of your body on the bottom of your left arm and gently grab on to the fingers of your left hand.

Now, take a nice slow deep breath in. As you exhale, gently apply pressure to the fingers of the left hand pressing them toward the front of your body; hold the stretch for a few seconds, then release.

Repeat for a total of eight repetitions. Do not over stretch.

7. Wrist and Forearm
Making a fist

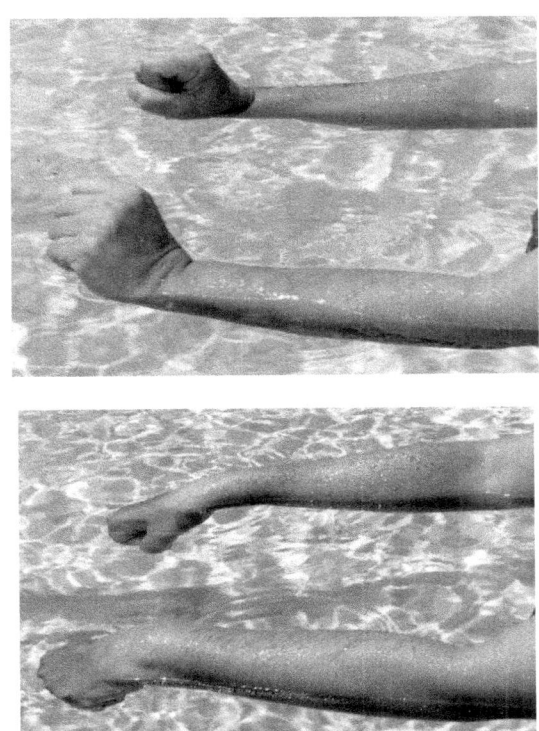

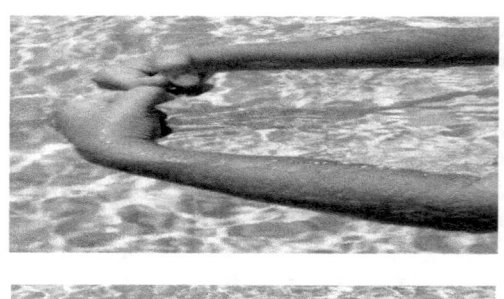

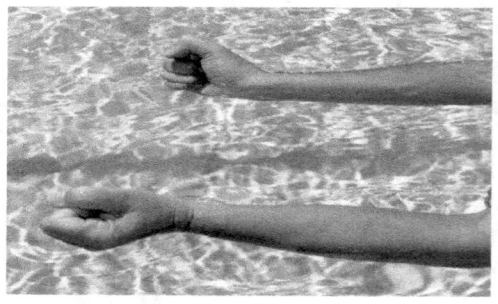

To Do:

You can put together the above wrist exercises in a unique way. Try performing these exercises with your hands closed in a fist. This will add a slight additional stretch to the muscles in the wrists and forearms. You can even add circles in one direction, repeat in the opposite position.

Warm ups for the Arms

1. Arms

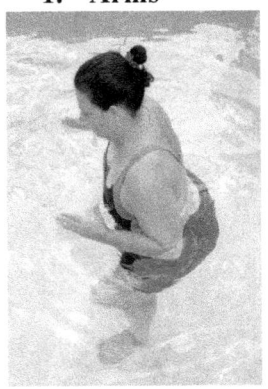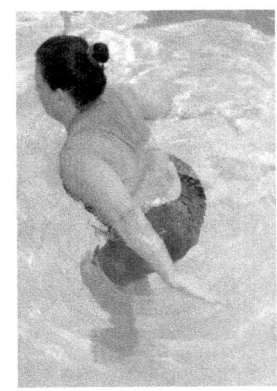

To Do:
Plant both of your feet flat on the bottom of the pool at shoulder width apart. Bend your knees and your elbows and bring your hands up towards you shoulders as shown in the picture above on the left. Your thumbs should be pointing towards your shoulders.

Slowly straighten your arms, bringing them through the water to as far back as you comfortably can, hold, and release back to starting point. Do a total of eight repetitions.

2. Arms and Shoulders

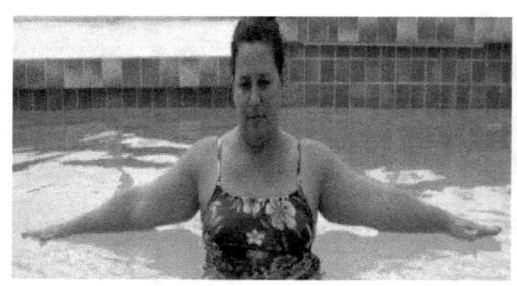

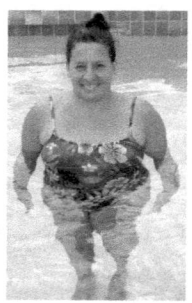

To Do:
Place your straight out from your sides. Bring your arms down into the water towards your side, hold, and release back to starting point. Do a total of eight repetitions.

4. Arms and Shoulders

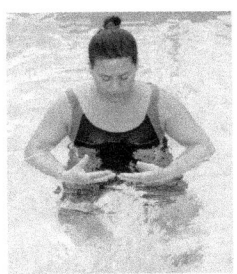

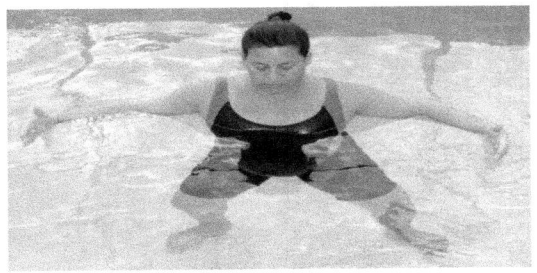

To Do:
Bend your knees and bring your hands in front and slowly pull your elbows backwards opening your chest, hold, and release back to starting point. Do a total of eight repetitions.

5. Arms and Shoulders

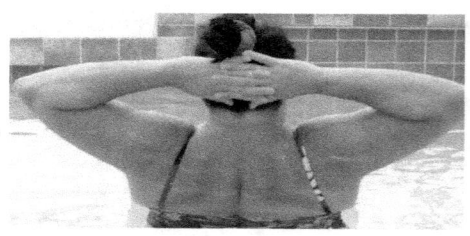

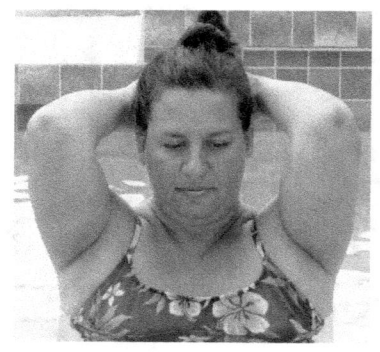

To Do:
Clasp your hands behind your head with elbows pointed outwards from the body as shown in the picture above. Slowly bring elbows towards the front of your body, hold, and release back to starting point. Do 8x's.

6. Arms and Shoulders

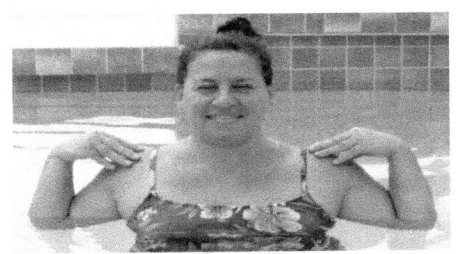

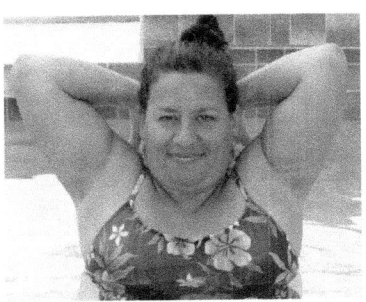

To Do:
Place your hands on your shoulder with elbows pointed downwards into the water as shown in the picture above.

Now, slowly bring elbows upwards pointing to the sky, hold, and release back to starting point. Do a total of eight repetitions.

7. Arms and Shoulders

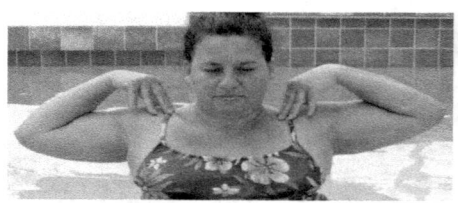

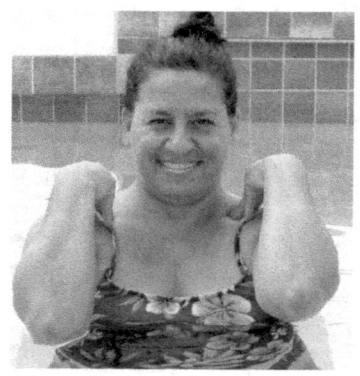

To Do:
Place your hands on your shoulder with elbows pointed outwards from your body as shown in the picture above. Slowly bring elbows in front of your body, hold, and release back to starting point. Do 8x's.

Warm ups---------Chest and Back

1.   Chest and Back

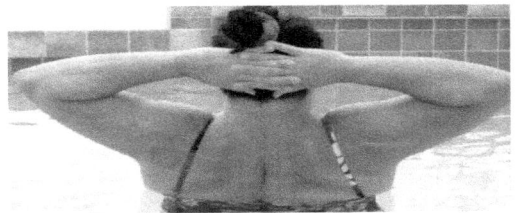

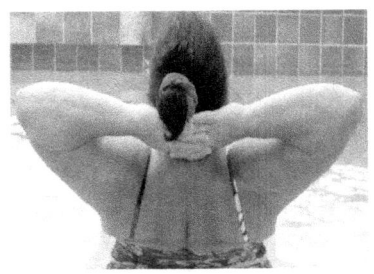

To Do:
Clasp your hands behind your head with elbows pointing away from your body as shown in the picture above. Slowly tilt your head backwards looking up at the sky, hold, and release back to starting point. Do 8x's.

2. Hip Sway

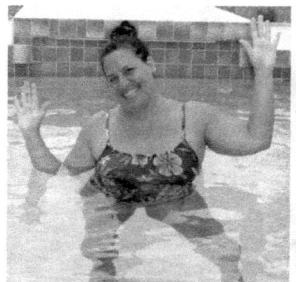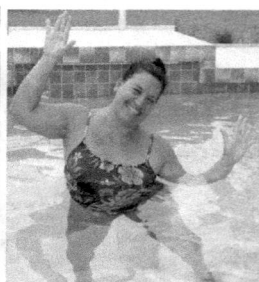

To Do:
With your feet on the bottom of the pool, swing hips from side to side. Have fun with this exercise. Pretend you are in Hawaii and move your hips to the right and then to the left in a smooth rhythm. You can add hip bumps or change the speed of your hip sways.

To have more fun, add exciting music and use your arms to sway to the music. Do pelvic tilts by pushing your pelvic girdle forward and backward.

Make circles in the water with your hips in one direction-then the other direction. Do eight repetitions.

Chapter Three
Basic Water Moves
- **Walking**
- **Knee-Ups**
- **Elbow to Knee**
- **Foot up in Front**
- **Foot up in Back**
- **Front Leg Ups**
- **Side Leg Lifts**
- **Inner/Outer Thigh**
- **Lunges**
- **Jumping Jacks**
- **Hamstring Curls**

1-Walking

Walking-Level One

Begin by walking forward and backward. Begin slowly just walking forward and backward. The faster you walk, the more intense the workout will be. In Level One you will try to keep the pace slow and steady so that you can keep your balance without too much stress on your body.

You can do this walking from the shallow to deeper waters or from one side of the pool to the other side and back.

Walking-Level Two
Walk at a faster pace. You can call it 'Power Walking' if you like. Move your arms through the water at your side as you try to walk briskly forward and backward. Don't overdo this exercise as it will tire you out and increase your heart rate very rapidly.

Walking-Level Three
Add power leaps and pushes off the bottom of the pool. Walk forward by pushing off the bottom of the pool and leaping forward.

Running in Place
Start running in place. Do this for 30 seconds working up to a minute or more. To add variety and intensity, practice running at different rates of speed for a great workout.

Running with Movement
Add running and direction. Run in a clockwise circle, then shift direction and run in a counterclockwise circle. Do this for several repetitions on each side.

2-Knee-Ups

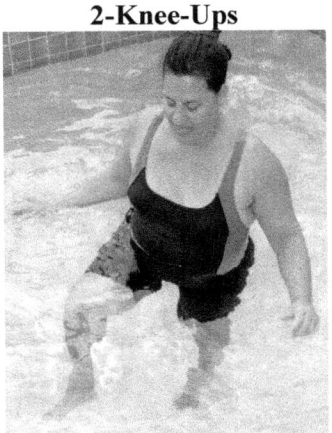

Knee-ups - Level One
Lift your right knee up as high as you can. (Do not go over a 90 degree angle). Press your right foot back to the bottom of the pool and straighten out your leg. Do this for a total of 8 repetitions and repeat the whole exercise on your left leg. Do 8 x's.

Knee-ups - Level Two
Increase the rate of speed that you are using to lift and lower each knee. The faster you can safely lift and lower your knee, the harder the workout will be.

Level Three
Alternate between lifting the right knee and lifting the left knee. The exercise will be "Right knee up, right knee down, Left knee up, left knee down." Do 16 repetitions. The faster you go, the more difficult the exercise.

2. Elbow to Knee

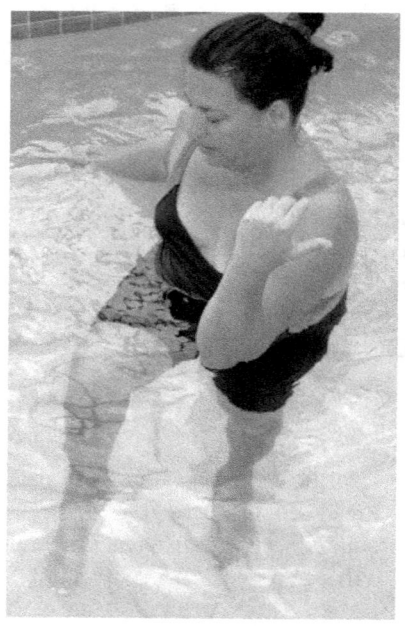

Level One
Lift your right knee up to the right of your body and bring your right elbow down to reach the right knee. Return the right foot back down to the bottom of the pool and straighten up your body. Do 8x's.

Level Two
Alternate the elbow to the opposite knee. The exercise will go like this: "Left elbow to right knee, straighten up, Right elbow to left knee, and straighten up. Do 16x's.

Level Three
Add speed and move forward and backward.

4. Touch Foot in Front

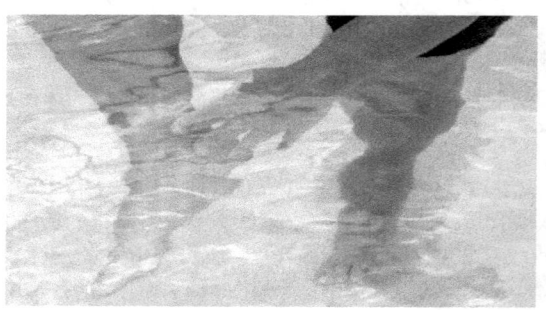

Level One
Bend your right knee and bring your right foot up in front of your body and you will reach down into the water with your left hand to touch the right foot. Straighten up and repeat again for at least 8 repetitions. Repeat on the other side. If you can't touch your foot that is alright-do what you can

Level Two
Add intensity by adding speed.

Level Three
Add speed and movement. You can move forward and backward while hoping from one foot to the other.

5. Touch Foot in Back

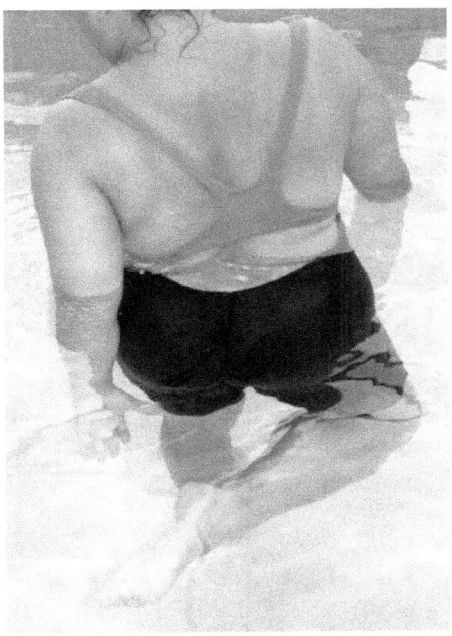

Level One
Bring your right foot up behind your body and reach down into the water with your left hand and try to touch your foot, straighten up your body. Repeat for 8 repetitions.

Level Two
Alternate left foot to right hand and right foot to left hand. The directions will be: "Left foot up, right hand down, Right foot up, left hand down." Repeat for 16x's.

To increase the intensity of this exercise even more, add speed to the movements. You will feel like you are hopping from one foot to the other.

Level Three
Add speed and movement. Move forward and backward while hopping from one foot to the other alternating reaching for your feet. The faster you go, the higher the intensity. Repeat for 16 to 25 repetitions.

6. Front Leg Lifts

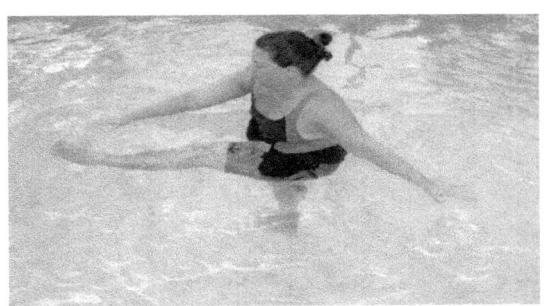

Level One
Inhale and bring your left leg straight up in front of you as high as you comfortably can, hold, and as you exhale bring your leg back to the starting position. Repeat 8x's. Repeat on other leg.

Level Two
Alternate lifting your left and right leg for a total of 16 repetitions.

Level Three
Add speed, hopping from right to left leg. Move forward and backward.

7. Side Leg Lifts

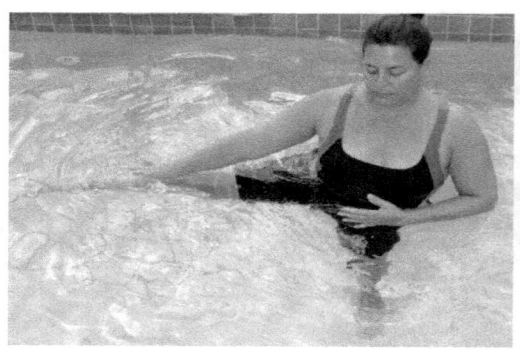

Level One
Inhale and lift your right leg straight up at your side as high as you can, exhale and release the leg back to the starting position. Do 8x's and repeat on other side.

Level Two
Alternate right and left side lifts. Do 16x's.

Level Three
Add movements forward and backward and side to side. Add speed to increase intensity.

8. Inner/Outer Thigh

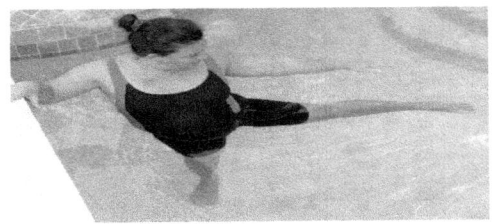

To Do: Inhale and lift your left leg out to the side of your body, hold, and as you exhale bring the leg back towards your body and sweep it front of your right leg.

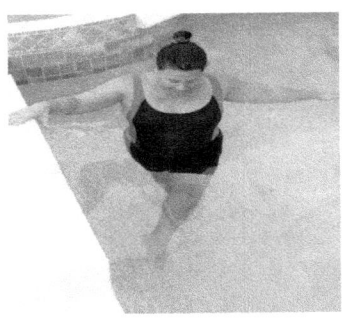

NOTE: Do not cross the midline of the body if you have had a hip replacement or other hip problems. Consult your doctor.

9. Lunges

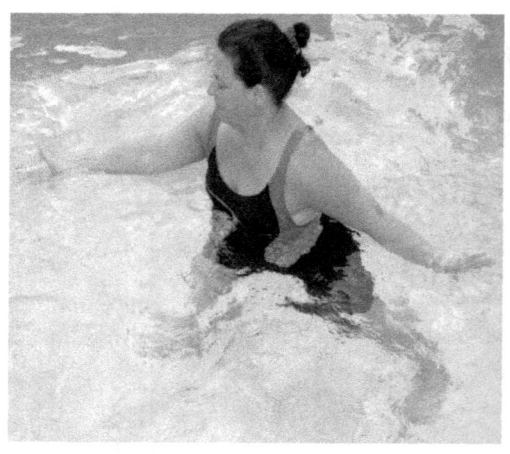

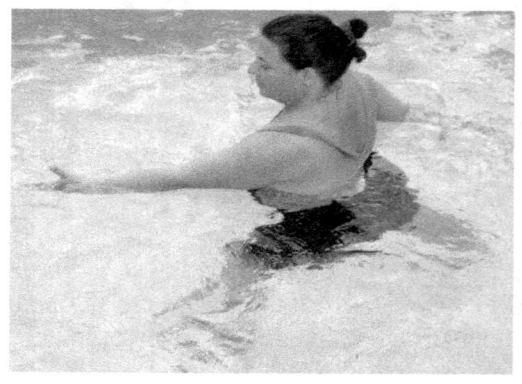

Level One
Jump up from the bottom of the pool; bring your right leg forward and your left leg back. As you land, your right foot should be in front of you and your left foot should be directly behind you. Now, jump up from the bottom of the pool again and this time bring your left foot in front of you and bring your right foot behind you. Do 16x's.

Level Two
Add speed.

Level Three
Add speed and movement.

10. Jumping Jacks

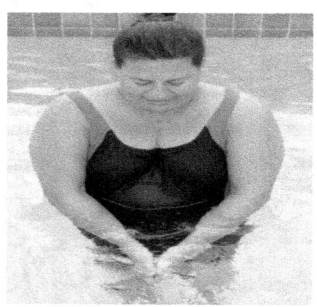

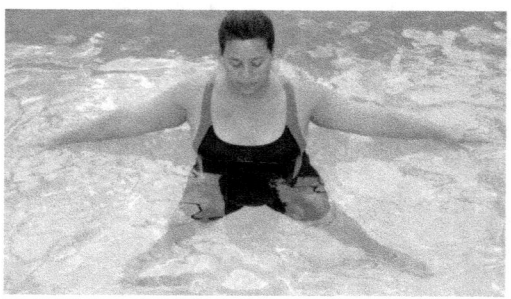

Level One
Bring both of your hands together in front of you and in the water. You will keep your hands IN the water throughout this entire exercise.

Inhale and jump up from the bottom of the pool and spread your legs out to both sides of your body. As you separate your legs, separate your arms out to your sides as well.

Exhale and jump up from the bottom of the pool and bring both of your legs and arms back together again as in the starting position above. Continue jumping out and in for a total of eight repetitions.

Level Two
Add speed and repetitions

Level Three
Add movement by doing jumping jacks to each of the four corners of the pool with a jump-turn to the next side.

You can also do this exercise in reverse by starting with legs apart and jump them together with a hop. Very intense.

11. Hamstring Curls

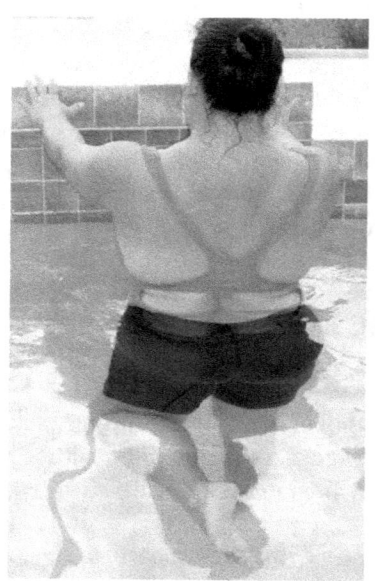

Level One
Inhale and bring the heel of your left up towards your left buttocks and down again. Do 8x's.

Level Two and Three
Alternate raising the left foot and right foot. 8x's Add speed and movement to increase the intensity of this exercise.

Chapter Four
Stretches

1. Shoulder Stretch

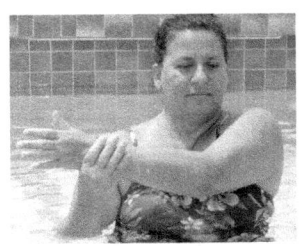

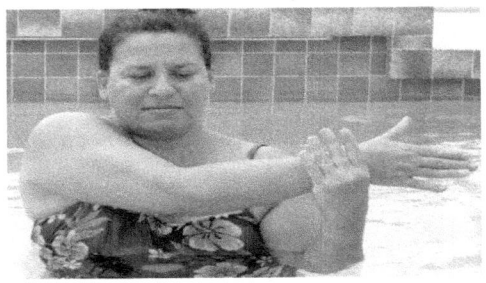

To Do:
Bring the left arm across the front of your body and gently grasp your left wrist with your right hand. Hold. Repeat on other side.

2. Shoulder Hug

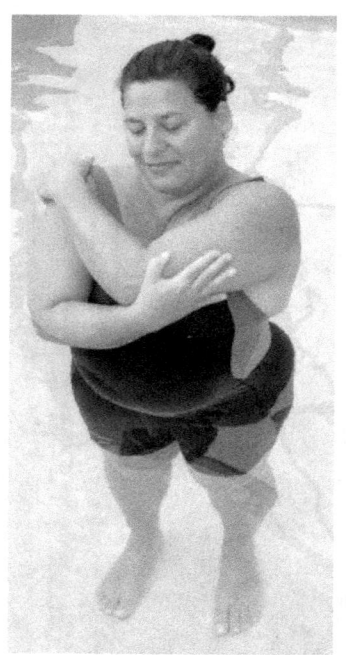

To Do:
Wrap your arms around each other and give yourself a big hug. Inhale and exhale freely and easily. Release your hug and switch your arms around and give yourself another big hug.

3. Tricep Stretch

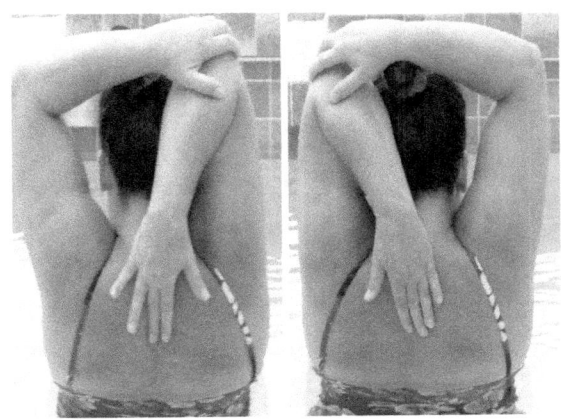

To Do:
Bend the elbow and bring the right hand down to lay flat on your back with the palm of your right hand on your back. Bring your left hand over and place it on your right elbow.

Gently add pressure to your right elbow to push it backward giving you a stretch in your triceps muscle. Breathe normally. Release and repeat on the other side. Do for a total of three repetitions.

4. Lat Stretch

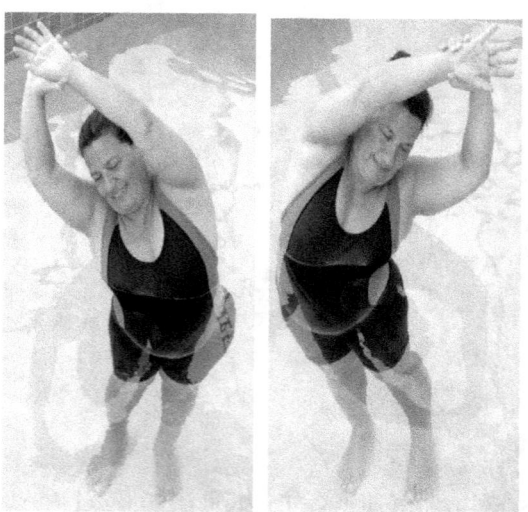

To Do:
Stand with feet flat on the bottom of the pool and shoulder width apart. Reach your left arm straight upward from your body. Inhale and clasp your left wrist with your right hand. As you exhale, gently pull the left hand, and arm, down towards the right. Inhale and return to starting position and exhale and release. Repeat on other side.

5. Hip Stretch

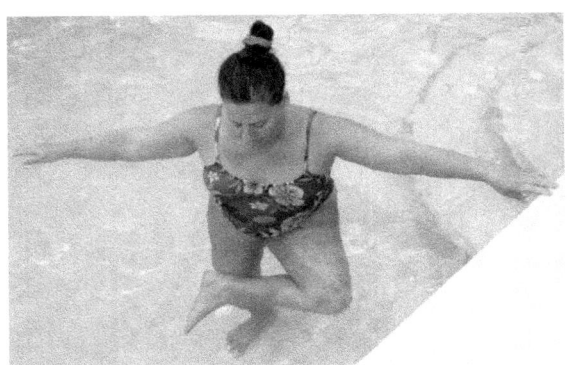

To Do:
Bend your left knee and bring your left up the front of your body and place it just above your knee.

Exhale, slowly bend your right knee and allow yourself to sink into the water as far as you can comfortably go. Hold, then release. Repeat this exercise on the other side using your right foot on your left thigh. To add more depth to this hip stretch exercise you can lift up off the heel of the foot on the bottom.

To add balance, do this exercise without holding on to the side of the pool.

4. Back Stretch

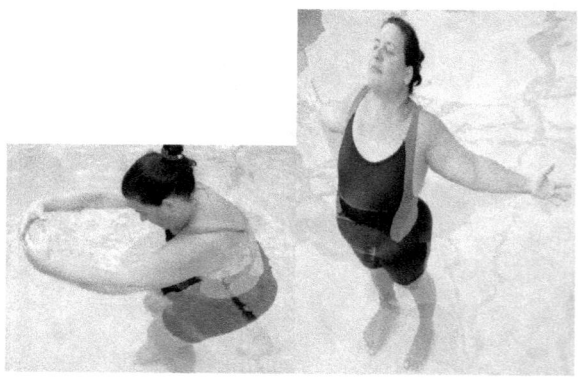

To Do:
Inhale, and as you exhale, bend your knees and slowly arch your back forward as shown in the first photo.

As you inhale, stand up straight and arch your back slightly backwards. Let your arms open wide from your sides opening up your chest as much as you comfortably can as shown in second photo.

When you exhale, roll yourself into the position as shown in the first photo. Repeat three times.

5. Side Stretch

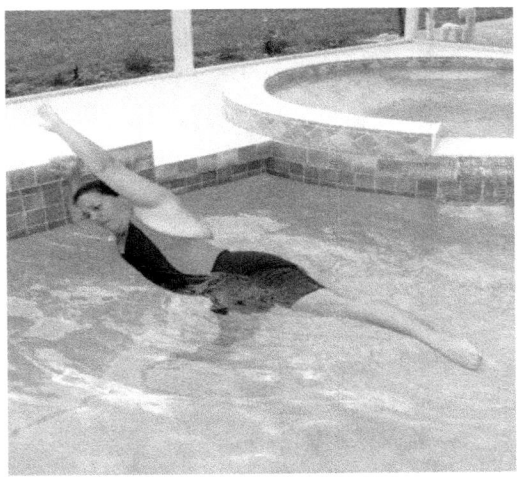

To Do:
Inhale and bend your right elbow, lifting your right arm straight upwards. As you exhale, bring the right arm over your head and lift your left leg straight out from the side of your body. Feel a good full body stretch, hold, and release back into starting position. Do 8 repetitions and repeat on opposite side.

6. Body Stretch

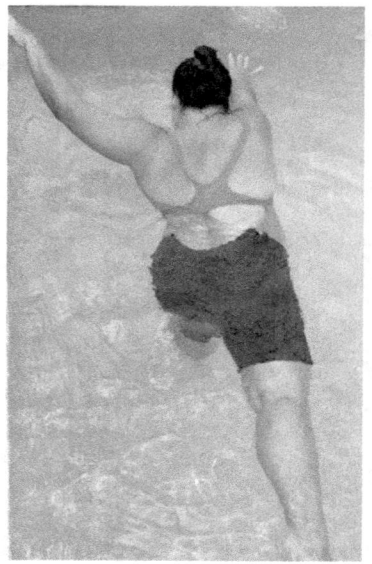

To Do: \Inhale and extend your right arm straight upwards. As you exhale, bend your torso and the right arm to the front as close to the top of the water line as you can get. Extend your right leg straight back behind you pointing your toes. Inhale and return to the starting position. Repeat this exercise on the other side.

Chapter Five
Balance

Balance-Yoga Style

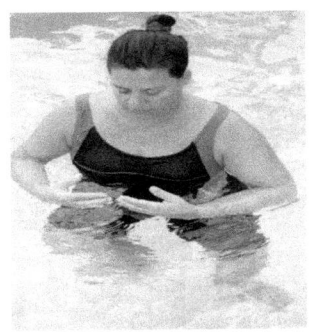

To Do: Bend both of your knees slightly outward at the sides. Bring both of your hands out in front of your body at just below heart level (should be just below the top of the water line).

The palms of both hands are facing in towards the front of your torso. Find a focal point and allow your mind to sit in that focal point. Inhale and exhale smoothly, slowly and deeply. Try to clear your mind of all outside annoyances and distractions.

Side Knee-Ups

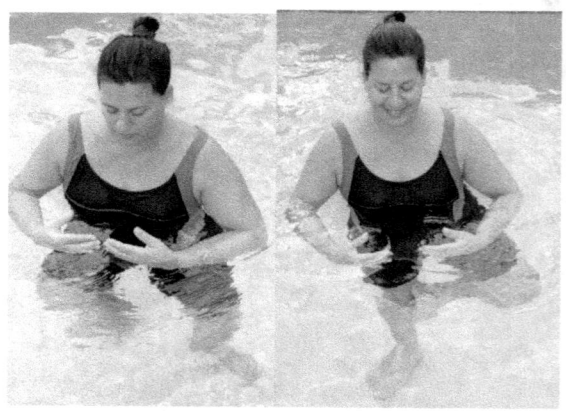

To Do:
Inhale and bend your left knee out to the side of your body and place the bottom of your left foot on the inside of your right leg just above the knee. Hold it there and breathe in and out slowly and without effort.

You may find that it is very difficult to keep your balance against the natural current of the water. Do your best.

When finished, release the foot to the starting position and repeat on the other side.

Do several times.

Balance Continued

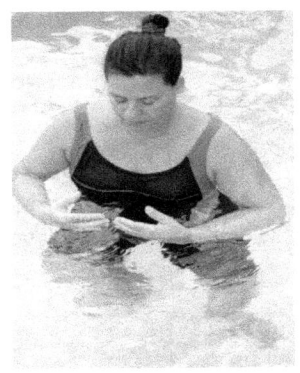

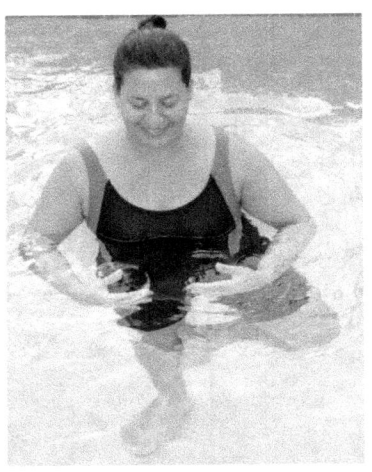

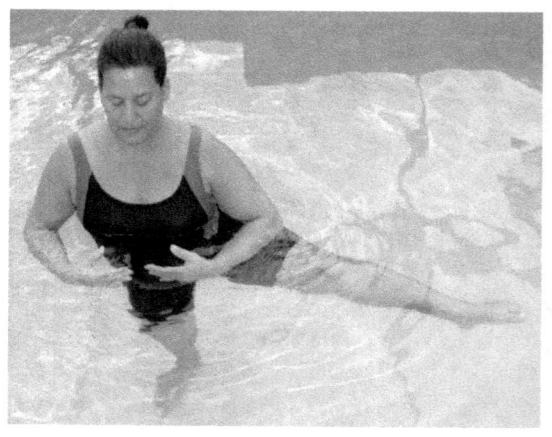

To Do:
Begin this exercise in the starting position. Bend your left knee and extend out to the side of your body and return to the starting position. Do eight repetitions and repeat on other side. Add breath work by doing the following:
"Inhale knee up-Exhale and extend the leg. Inhale knee bends. Exhale and return leg to bottom of pool."

Cool Down

Cool downs are a series of movements that are used after an exercise class as a means to return the heart rate back to its normal pre-exercise rate.

If completing all the exercises in this book at one time is too much for you, then pick one exercise for the ankles, one exercise for the legs, etc. and then just do those exercises for a week, or month, as the case may be. You could then add, or trade out, the exercises for the following workout period.

The Qi Ball

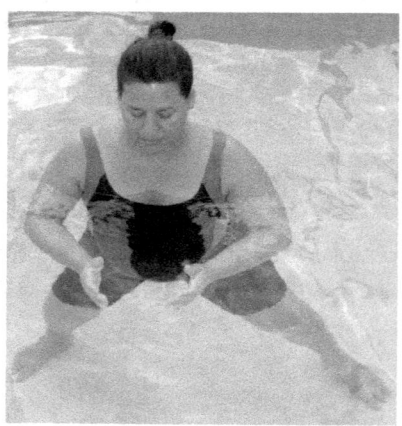

To Do:

Stand with your feet firmly planted on the bottom of the pool. Bring both of your hands up in front of your body at heart level (should be just under the water line) with palms facing each other.

Inhale and pull the hands away from each other to about 1-2' apart. When you exhale, bring the hands towards each other to about 6-12" apart. Continue inhaling and exhaling in the way for as long as you enjoy this exercise.

www.ingramcontent.com/pod-product-compliance
Lightning Source LLC
Chambersburg PA
CBHW062109280526
45788CB00003B/1402